Paranormal Investigation

This book belongs to:

_____

Investigation Date _____   Time _____

Address _____

Haunt Information

What happens?
Date of first experience
Description of events

Suspected entity information

Possible Names	Dates alive
Where entity lived	Entity's motives/wants
Story	

Investigation recordings

Site Temperature										
	Cold				Neutral					Hot
Atmosphere										
	Oppressive				Neutral					Light
Site observation										
Sensory Notes										

Equipment Used

Equipment	Readings

Investigation Date _____   Time _____

Address _____

Haunt Information

What happens?
Date of first experience
Description of events

Suspected entity information

Possible Names	Dates alive
Where entity lived	Entity's motives/wants
Story	

Investigation recordings

Site Temperature	Cold — Neutral — Hot
Atmosphere	Oppressive — Neutral — Light
Site observation	
Sensory Notes	

Equipment Used

Equipment	Readings

Investigation Date _____   Time _____

Address _____

Haunt Information

What happens?
Date of first experience
Description of events

Suspected entity information

Possible Names	Dates alive
Where entity lived	Entity's motives/wants
Story	

Investigation recordings

Site Temperature	Cold · · · · Neutral · · · · Hot	
Atmosphere	Oppressive · · · · Neutral · · · · Light	
Site observation		
Sensory Notes		

Equipment Used

Equipment	Readings

Investigation Date _____ Time _____

Address _____

Haunt Information

What happens?
Date of first experience
Description of events

Suspected entity information

Possible Names	Dates alive
Where entity lived	Entity's motives/wants
Story	

Investigation recordings

Site Temperature									
	Cold				Neutral				Hot
Atmosphere									
	Oppressive				Neutral				Light
Site observation									
Sensory Notes									

Equipment Used

Equipment	Readings

Investigation Date _____ Time _____

Address _____

Haunt Information

What happens?
Date of first experience
Description of events

Suspected entity information

Possible Names	Dates alive
Where entity lived	Entity's motives/wants
Story	

Investigation recordings

Site Temperature										
	Cold				Neutral					Hot
Atmosphere										
	Oppressive				Neutral					Light

Site observation

Sensory Notes

Equipment Used

Equipment	Readings

Investigation Date _____   Time _____

Address _____

Haunt Information

What happens?
Date of first experience
Description of events

Suspected entity information

Possible Names	Dates alive
Where entity lived	Entity's motives/wants
Story	

Investigation recordings

Site Temperature		
	Cold — Neutral — Hot	
Atmosphere		
	Oppressive — Neutral — Light	
Site observation		
Sensory Notes		

Equipment Used

Equipment	Readings

Investigation Date _____   Time _____

Address _____

Haunt Information

What happens?
Date of first experience
Description of events

Suspected entity information

Possible Names	Dates alive
Where entity lived	Entity's motives/wants
Story	

Investigation recordings

Site Temperature	Cold · · · · Neutral · · · · Hot	
Atmosphere	Oppressive · · · · Neutral · · · · Light	
Site observation		
Sensory Notes		

Equipment Used

Equipment	Readings

Investigation Date _____   Time _____

Address _____

Haunt Information

What happens?
Date of first experience
Description of events

Suspected entity information

Possible Names	Dates alive
Where entity lived	Entity's motives/wants
Story	

Investigation recordings

Site Temperature	Cold — Neutral — Hot
Atmosphere	Oppressive — Neutral — Light
Site observation	
Sensory Notes	

Equipment Used

Equipment	Readings

Investigation Date _____   Time _____

Address _____

Haunt Information

What happens?
Date of first experience
Description of events

Suspected entity information

Possible Names	Dates alive
Where entity lived	Entity's motives/wants
Story	

Investigation recordings

Site Temperature	Cold — Neutral — Hot
Atmosphere	Oppressive — Neutral — Light
Site observation	
Sensory Notes	

Equipment Used

Equipment	Readings

Investigation Date _____   Time _____

Address _____

Haunt Information

What happens?
Date of first experience
Description of events

Suspected entity information

Possible Names	Dates alive
Where entity lived	Entity's motives/wants
Story	

Investigation recordings

Site Temperature	Cold	Neutral	Hot
Atmosphere	Oppressive	Neutral	Light
Site observation			
Sensory Notes			

Equipment Used

Equipment	Readings

Investigation Date _____   Time _____

Address _____

Haunt Information

What happens?
Date of first experience
Description of events

Suspected entity information

Possible Names	Dates alive
Where entity lived	Entity's motives/wants
Story	

Investigation recordings

Site Temperature									
	Cold				Neutral				Hot
Atmosphere									
	Oppressive				Neutral				Light
Site observation									
Sensory Notes									

Equipment Used

Equipment	Readings

Investigation Date _____   Time _____

Address _____

Haunt Information

What happens?
Date of first experience
Description of events

Suspected entity information

Possible Names	Dates alive
Where entity lived	Entity's motives/wants
Story	

Investigation recordings

Site Temperature										
	Cold				Neutral					Hot
Atmosphere										
	Oppressive				Neutral					Light
Site observation										
Sensory Notes										

Equipment Used

Equipment	Readings

Investigation Date _____   Time _____

Address _____

Haunt Information

What happens?
Date of first experience
Description of events

Suspected entity information

Possible Names	Dates alive
Where entity lived	Entity's motives/wants
Story	

Investigation recordings

Site Temperature									
	Cold				Neutral				Hot
Atmosphere									
	Oppressive				Neutral				Light

Site observation

Sensory Notes

Equipment Used

Equipment	Readings

Investigation Date _____   Time _____

Address _____

Haunt Information

What happens?
Date of first experience
Description of events

Suspected entity information

Possible Names	Dates alive
Where entity lived	Entity's motives/wants
Story	

Investigation recordings

Site Temperature										
	Cold				Neutral					Hot
Atmosphere										
	Oppressive				Neutral					Light
Site observation										
Sensory Notes										

Equipment Used

Equipment	Readings

Investigation Date _____   Time _____

Address _____

Haunt Information

What happens?
Date of first experience
Description of events

Suspected entity information

Possible Names	Dates alive
Where entity lived	Entity's motives/wants
Story	

Investigation recordings

Site Temperature	Cold — Neutral — Hot
Atmosphere	Oppressive — Neutral — Light
Site observation	
Sensory Notes	

Equipment Used

Equipment	Readings

Investigation Date _____   Time _____

Address _____

Haunt Information

What happens?
Date of first experience
Description of events

Suspected entity information

Possible Names	Dates alive
Where entity lived	Entity's motives/wants
Story	

Investigation recordings

Site Temperature	Cold — Neutral — Hot	
Atmosphere	Oppressive — Neutral — Light	
Site observation		
Sensory Notes		

Equipment Used

Equipment	Readings

Investigation Date _____   Time _____

Address _____

Haunt Information

What happens?
Date of first experience
Description of events

Suspected entity information

Possible Names	Dates alive
Where entity lived	Entity's motives/wants
Story	

Investigation recordings

Site Temperature	Cold — Neutral — Hot	
Atmosphere	Oppressive — Neutral — Light	
Site observation		
Sensory Notes		

Equipment Used

Equipment	Readings

Investigation Date _____   Time _____

Address _____

Haunt Information

What happens?
Date of first experience
Description of events

Suspected entity information

Possible Names	Dates alive
Where entity lived	Entity's motives/wants
Story	

Investigation recordings

Site Temperature	Cold — Neutral — Hot
Atmosphere	Oppressive — Neutral — Light
Site observation	
Sensory Notes	

Equipment Used

Equipment	Readings

Investigation Date _____   Time _____

Address _____

Haunt Information

What happens?
Date of first experience
Description of events

Suspected entity information

Possible Names	Dates alive
Where entity lived	Entity's motives/wants
Story	

Investigation recordings

Site Temperature										
	Cold				Neutral					Hot
Atmosphere										
	Oppressive				Neutral					Light

Site observation

Sensory Notes

Equipment Used

Equipment	Readings

Investigation Date _____   Time _____

Address _____

Haunt Information

What happens?
Date of first experience
Description of events

Suspected entity information

Possible Names	Dates alive
Where entity lived	Entity's motives/wants
Story	

Investigation recordings

Site Temperature	Cold — Neutral — Hot	
Atmosphere	Oppressive — Neutral — Light	
Site observation		
Sensory Notes		

Equipment Used

Equipment	Readings

Investigation Date _____   Time _____

Address _____

Haunt Information

What happens?
Date of first experience
Description of events

Suspected entity information

Possible Names	Dates alive
Where entity lived	Entity's motives/wants
Story	

Investigation recordings

Site Temperature									
	Cold				Neutral				Hot
Atmosphere									
	Oppressive				Neutral				Light
Site observation									
Sensory Notes									

Equipment Used

Equipment	Readings

Investigation Date _____   Time _____

Address _____

Haunt Information

What happens?
Date of first experience
Description of events

Suspected entity information

Possible Names	Dates alive
Where entity lived	Entity's motives/wants
Story	

Investigation recordings

Site Temperature									
	Cold				Neutral				Hot
Atmosphere									
	Oppressive				Neutral				Light
Site observation									
Sensory Notes									

Equipment Used

Equipment	Readings

Investigation Date _____   Time _____

Address _____

Haunt Information

What happens?
Date of first experience
Description of events

Suspected entity information

Possible Names	Dates alive
Where entity lived	Entity's motives/wants
Story	

Investigation recordings

Site Temperature										
	Cold				Neutral					Hot
Atmosphere										
	Oppressive				Neutral					Light
Site observation										
Sensory Notes										

Equipment Used

Equipment	Readings

Investigation Date _____   Time _____

Address _____

Haunt Information

What happens?
Date of first experience
Description of events

Suspected entity information

Possible Names	Dates alive
Where entity lived	Entity's motives/wants
Story	

Investigation recordings

Site Temperature	Cold — Neutral — Hot
Atmosphere	Oppressive — Neutral — Light
Site observation	
Sensory Notes	

Equipment Used

Equipment	Readings

Investigation Date _____   Time _____

Address _____

Haunt Information

What happens?
Date of first experience
Description of events

Suspected entity information

Possible Names	Dates alive
Where entity lived	Entity's motives/wants
Story	

Investigation recordings

Site Temperature	Cold — Neutral — Hot
Atmosphere	Oppressive — Neutral — Light
Site observation	
Sensory Notes	

Equipment Used

Equipment	Readings

Investigation Date _____   Time _____

Address _____

Haunt Information

What happens?
Date of first experience
Description of events

Suspected entity information

Possible Names	Dates alive
Where entity lived	Entity's motives/wants
Story	

Investigation recordings

Site Temperature		
	Cold — Neutral — Hot	
Atmosphere		
	Oppressive — Neutral — Light	
Site observation		
Sensory Notes		

Equipment Used

Equipment	Readings

Investigation Date _____   Time _____

Address _____

Haunt Information

What happens?
Date of first experience
Description of events

Suspected entity information

Possible Names	Dates alive
Where entity lived	Entity's motives/wants
Story	

Investigation recordings

Site Temperature									
	Cold				Neutral				Hot
Atmosphere									
	Oppressive				Neutral				Light
Site observation									
Sensory Notes									

Equipment Used

Equipment	Readings

Investigation Date _____ Time _____

Address _____

Haunt Information

What happens?
Date of first experience
Description of events

Suspected entity information

Possible Names	Dates alive
Where entity lived	Entity's motives/wants
Story	

Investigation recordings

Site Temperature								
	Cold				Neutral			Hot
Atmosphere								
	Oppressive				Neutral			Light

Site observation

Sensory Notes

Equipment Used

Equipment	Readings

Investigation Date _____   Time _____

Address _____

Haunt Information

What happens?
Date of first experience
Description of events

Suspected entity information

Possible Names	Dates alive
Where entity lived	Entity's motives/wants
Story	

Investigation recordings

Site Temperature										
	Cold				Neutral					Hot
Atmosphere										
	Oppressive				Neutral					Light
Site observation										
Sensory Notes										

Equipment Used

Equipment	Readings

Investigation Date _____   Time _____

Address _____

Haunt Information

What happens?
Date of first experience
Description of events

Suspected entity information

Possible Names	Dates alive
Where entity lived	Entity's motives/wants
Story	

Investigation recordings

Site Temperature										
	Cold				Neutral					Hot
Atmosphere										
	Oppressive				Neutral					Light
Site observation										
Sensory Notes										

Equipment Used

Equipment	Readings

Investigation Date _____   Time _____

Address _____

Haunt Information

What happens?
Date of first experience
Description of events

Suspected entity information

Possible Names	Dates alive
Where entity lived	Entity's motives/wants
Story	

Investigation recordings

Site Temperature	Cold — Neutral — Hot
Atmosphere	Oppressive — Neutral — Light
Site observation	
Sensory Notes	

Equipment Used

Equipment	Readings

Investigation Date _____   Time _____

Address _____

Haunt Information

What happens?
Date of first experience
Description of events

Suspected entity information

Possible Names	Dates alive
Where entity lived	Entity's motives/wants
Story	

Investigation recordings

Site Temperature	Cold — Neutral — Hot
Atmosphere	Oppressive — Neutral — Light
Site observation	
Sensory Notes	

Equipment Used

Equipment	Readings

Investigation Date _____ Time _____

Address _____

Haunt Information

What happens?
Date of first experience
Description of events

Suspected entity information

Possible Names	Dates alive
Where entity lived	Entity's motives/wants
Story	

Investigation recordings

Site Temperature										
	Cold				Neutral					Hot
Atmosphere										
	Oppressive				Neutral					Light
Site observation										
Sensory Notes										

Equipment Used

Equipment	Readings

Investigation Date _____   Time _____

Address _____

Haunt Information

What happens?
Date of first experience
Description of events

Suspected entity information

Possible Names	Dates alive
Where entity lived	Entity's motives/wants
Story	

Investigation recordings

Site Temperature									
	Cold				Neutral				Hot
Atmosphere									
	Oppressive				Neutral				Light
Site observation									
Sensory Notes									

Equipment Used

Equipment	Readings

Investigation Date _____   Time _____

Address _____

Haunt Information

What happens?
Date of first experience
Description of events

Suspected entity information

Possible Names	Dates alive
Where entity lived	Entity's motives/wants
Story	

Investigation recordings

Site Temperature

Cold   Neutral   Hot

Atmosphere

Oppressive   Neutral   Light

Site observation

Sensory Notes

Equipment Used

Equipment	Readings

Investigation Date _____   Time _____

Address _____

Haunt Information

What happens?
Date of first experience
Description of events

Suspected entity information

Possible Names	Dates alive
Where entity lived	Entity's motives/wants
Story	

Investigation recordings

Site Temperature	Cold — Neutral — Hot
Atmosphere	Oppressive — Neutral — Light
Site observation	
Sensory Notes	

Equipment Used

Equipment	Readings

Investigation Date _____   Time _____

Address _____

Haunt Information

What happens?
Date of first experience
Description of events

Suspected entity information

Possible Names	Dates alive
Where entity lived	Entity's motives/wants
Story	

Investigation recordings

Site Temperature	Cold — Neutral — Hot
Atmosphere	Oppressive — Neutral — Light
Site observation	
Sensory Notes	

Equipment Used

Equipment	Readings

Investigation Date _____ Time _____

Address _____

Haunt Information

What happens?
Date of first experience
Description of events

Suspected entity information

Possible Names	Dates alive
Where entity lived	Entity's motives/wants
Story	

Investigation recordings

Site Temperature									
	Cold				Neutral				Hot

Atmosphere									
	Oppressive				Neutral				Light

Site observation

Sensory Notes

Equipment Used

Equipment	Readings

Investigation Date _____   Time _____

Address _____

Haunt Information

What happens?
Date of first experience
Description of events

Suspected entity information

Possible Names	Dates alive
Where entity lived	Entity's motives/wants
Story	

Investigation recordings

Site Temperature	Cold — Neutral — Hot
Atmosphere	Oppressive — Neutral — Light
Site observation	
Sensory Notes	

Equipment Used

Equipment	Readings

Investigation Date _____ Time _____

Address _____

Haunt Information

What happens?
Date of first experience
Description of events

Suspected entity information

Possible Names	Dates alive
Where entity lived	Entity's motives/wants
Story	

Investigation recordings

Site Temperature										
	Cold				Neutral					Hot
Atmosphere										
	Oppressive				Neutral					Light
Site observation										
Sensory Notes										

Equipment Used

Equipment	Readings

Investigation Date _____   Time _____

Address _____

Haunt Information

What happens?
Date of first experience
Description of events

Suspected entity information

Possible Names	Dates alive
Where entity lived	Entity's motives/wants
Story	

Investigation recordings

Site Temperature	Cold — Neutral — Hot	
Atmosphere	Oppressive — Neutral — Light	
Site observation		
Sensory Notes		

Equipment Used

Equipment	Readings

Investigation Date _____   Time _____

Address _____

Haunt Information

What happens?
Date of first experience
Description of events

Suspected entity information

Possible Names	Dates alive
Where entity lived	Entity's motives/wants
Story	

Investigation recordings

Site Temperature	Cold — Neutral — Hot
Atmosphere	Oppressive — Neutral — Light
Site observation	
Sensory Notes	

Equipment Used

Equipment	Readings

Investigation Date _____   Time _____

Address _____

Haunt Information

What happens?
Date of first experience
Description of events

Suspected entity information

Possible Names	Dates alive
Where entity lived	Entity's motives/wants
Story	

Investigation recordings

Site Temperature	Cold — Neutral — Hot
Atmosphere	Oppressive — Neutral — Light
Site observation	
Sensory Notes	

Equipment Used

Equipment	Readings

Investigation Date _____   Time _____

Address _____

Haunt Information

What happens?
Date of first experience
Description of events

Suspected entity information

Possible Names	Dates alive
Where entity lived	Entity's motives/wants
Story	

Investigation recordings

Site Temperature	Cold	Neutral	Hot
Atmosphere	Oppressive	Neutral	Light
Site observation			
Sensory Notes			

Equipment Used

Equipment	Readings

Investigation Date _____ Time _____

Address _____

Haunt Information

What happens?
Date of first experience
Description of events

Suspected entity information

Possible Names	Dates alive
Where entity lived	Entity's motives/wants
Story	

Investigation recordings

Site Temperature										
	Cold				Neutral					Hot
Atmosphere										
	Oppressive				Neutral					Light
Site observation										
Sensory Notes										

Equipment Used

Equipment	Readings

Investigation Date _____   Time _____

Address _____

Haunt Information

What happens?
Date of first experience
Description of events

Suspected entity information

Possible Names	Dates alive
Where entity lived	Entity's motives/wants
Story	

Investigation recordings

Site Temperature	Cold — Neutral — Hot
Atmosphere	Oppressive — Neutral — Light
Site observation	
Sensory Notes	

Equipment Used

Equipment	Readings

Investigation Date _____ Time _____

Address _____

Haunt Information

What happens?
Date of first experience
Description of events

Suspected entity information

Possible Names	Dates alive
Where entity lived	Entity's motives/wants
Story	

Investigation recordings

Site Temperature									
	Cold				Neutral				Hot
Atmosphere									
	Oppressive				Neutral				Light

Site observation

Sensory Notes

Equipment Used

Equipment	Readings

Investigation Date _____ Time _____

Address _____

Haunt Information

What happens?
Date of first experience
Description of events

Suspected entity information

Possible Names	Dates alive
Where entity lived	Entity's motives/wants
Story	

Investigation recordings

Site Temperature	Cold — Neutral — Hot
Atmosphere	Oppressive — Neutral — Light
Site observation	
Sensory Notes	

Equipment Used

Equipment	Readings

Investigation Date _____   Time _____

Address _____

Haunt Information

What happens?
Date of first experience
Description of events

Suspected entity information

Possible Names	Dates alive
Where entity lived	Entity's motives/wants
Story	

Investigation recordings

Site Temperature	Cold — Neutral — Hot	
Atmosphere	Oppressive — Neutral — Light	
Site observation		
Sensory Notes		

Equipment Used

Equipment	Readings

Investigation Date _____   Time _____

Address _____

Haunt Information

What happens?
Date of first experience
Description of events

Suspected entity information

Possible Names	Dates alive
Where entity lived	Entity's motives/wants
Story	

Investigation recordings

Site Temperature	Cold	Neutral	Hot
Atmosphere	Oppressive	Neutral	Light
Site observation			
Sensory Notes			

Equipment Used

Equipment	Readings

Investigation Date _____   Time _____

Address _____

Haunt Information

What happens?
Date of first experience
Description of events

Suspected entity information

Possible Names	Dates alive
Where entity lived	Entity's motives/wants
Story	

Investigation recordings

Site Temperature										
	Cold				Neutral					Hot
Atmosphere										
	Oppressive				Neutral					Light
Site observation										
Sensory Notes										

Equipment Used

Equipment	Readings

Investigation Date _____   Time _____

Address _____

Haunt Information

What happens?
Date of first experience
Description of events

Suspected entity information

Possible Names	Dates alive
Where entity lived	Entity's motives/wants
Story	

Investigation recordings

Site Temperature									
	Cold				Neutral				Hot
Atmosphere									
	Oppressive				Neutral				Light
Site observation									
Sensory Notes									

Equipment Used

Equipment	Readings

Investigation Date _____   Time _____

Address _____

Haunt Information

What happens?
Date of first experience
Description of events

Suspected entity information

Possible Names	Dates alive
Where entity lived	Entity's motives/wants
Story	

Investigation recordings

Site Temperature	Cold — Neutral — Hot	
Atmosphere	Oppressive — Neutral — Light	
Site observation		
Sensory Notes		

Equipment Used

Equipment	Readings

Investigation Date _____   Time _____

Address _____

Haunt Information

What happens?
Date of first experience
Description of events

Suspected entity information

Possible Names	Dates alive
Where entity lived	Entity's motives/wants
Story	

Investigation recordings

Site Temperature	Cold — Neutral — Hot	
Atmosphere	Oppressive — Neutral — Light	
Site observation		
Sensory Notes		

Equipment Used

Equipment	Readings

Investigation Date _____   Time _____

Address _____

Haunt Information

What happens?
Date of first experience
Description of events

Suspected entity information

Possible Names	Dates alive
Where entity lived	Entity's motives/wants
Story	

Investigation recordings

Site Temperature									
	Cold				Neutral				Hot
Atmosphere									
	Oppressive				Neutral				Light
Site observation									
Sensory Notes									

Equipment Used

Equipment	Readings

Investigation Date _____   Time _____

Address _____

Haunt Information

What happens?
Date of first experience
Description of events

Suspected entity information

Possible Names	Dates alive
Where entity lived	Entity's motives/wants
Story	

Investigation recordings

Site Temperature

Cold · Neutral · Hot

Atmosphere

Oppressive · Neutral · Light

Site observation

Sensory Notes

Equipment Used

Equipment	Readings

Investigation Date _____   Time _____

Address _____

Haunt Information

What happens?
Date of first experience
Description of events

Suspected entity information

Possible Names	Dates alive
Where entity lived	Entity's motives/wants
Story	

Investigation recordings

Site Temperature	Cold — Neutral — Hot
Atmosphere	Oppressive — Neutral — Light
Site observation	
Sensory Notes	

Equipment Used

Equipment	Readings

Investigation Date _____   Time _____

Address _____

Haunt Information

What happens?
Date of first experience
Description of events

Suspected entity information

Possible Names	Dates alive
Where entity lived	Entity's motives/wants
Story	

Investigation recordings

Site Temperature										
	Cold				Neutral					Hot
Atmosphere										
	Oppressive				Neutral					Light
Site observation										
Sensory Notes										

Equipment Used

Equipment	Readings

Investigation Date _____   Time _____

Address _____

Haunt Information

What happens?
Date of first experience
Description of events

Suspected entity information

Possible Names	Dates alive
Where entity lived	Entity's motives/wants
Story	

Investigation recordings

Site Temperature		
	Cold — Neutral — Hot	
Atmosphere		
	Oppressive — Neutral — Light	
Site observation		
Sensory Notes		

Equipment Used

Equipment	Readings

Investigation Date _____   Time _____

Address _____

Haunt Information

What happens?
Date of first experience
Description of events

Suspected entity information

Possible Names	Dates alive
Where entity lived	Entity's motives/wants
Story	

Investigation recordings

Site Temperature	Cold — Neutral — Hot
Atmosphere	Oppressive — Neutral — Light
Site observation	
Sensory Notes	

Equipment Used

Equipment	Readings

Investigation Date _____   Time _____

Address _____

Haunt Information

What happens?
Date of first experience
Description of events

Suspected entity information

Possible Names	Dates alive
Where entity lived	Entity's motives/wants
Story	

Investigation recordings

Site Temperature	Cold — Neutral — Hot
Atmosphere	Oppressive — Neutral — Light
Site observation	
Sensory Notes	

Equipment Used

Equipment	Readings

Investigation Date _____ Time _____

Address _____

Haunt Information

What happens?
Date of first experience
Description of events

Suspected entity information

Possible Names	Dates alive
Where entity lived	Entity's motives/wants
Story	

Investigation recordings

Site Temperature									
	Cold				Neutral				Hot
Atmosphere									
	Oppressive				Neutral				Light
Site observation									
Sensory Notes									

Equipment Used

Equipment	Readings

Investigation Date _____   Time _____

Address _____

Haunt Information

What happens?
Date of first experience
Description of events

Suspected entity information

Possible Names	Dates alive
Where entity lived	Entity's motives/wants
Story	

Investigation recordings

Site Temperature	Cold — Neutral — Hot
Atmosphere	Oppressive — Neutral — Light
Site observation	
Sensory Notes	

Equipment Used

Equipment	Readings

Investigation Date _____   Time _____

Address _____

Haunt Information

What happens?
Date of first experience
Description of events

Suspected entity information

Possible Names	Dates alive
Where entity lived	Entity's motives/wants
Story	

Investigation recordings

Site Temperature	Cold — Neutral — Hot
Atmosphere	Oppressive — Neutral — Light
Site observation	
Sensory Notes	

Equipment Used

Equipment	Readings

Investigation Date _____ Time _____

Address _____

Haunt Information

What happens?
Date of first experience
Description of events

Suspected entity information

Possible Names	Dates alive
Where entity lived	Entity's motives/wants
Story	

Investigation recordings

Site Temperature										
	Cold				Neutral					Hot
Atmosphere										
	Oppressive				Neutral					Light
Site observation										
Sensory Notes										

Equipment Used

Equipment	Readings

Investigation Date _____   Time _____

Address _____

Haunt Information

What happens?
Date of first experience
Description of events

Suspected entity information

Possible Names	Dates alive
Where entity lived	Entity's motives/wants
Story	

Investigation recordings

Site Temperature	Cold ⬚⬚⬚⬚⬚⬚⬚⬚⬚ Hot	Neutral
Atmosphere	Oppressive ⬚⬚⬚⬚⬚⬚⬚⬚⬚ Light	Neutral
Site observation		
Sensory Notes		

Equipment Used

Equipment	Readings

Investigation Date _____   Time _____

Address _____

Haunt Information

What happens?
Date of first experience
Description of events

Suspected entity information

Possible Names	Dates alive
Where entity lived	Entity's motives/wants
Story	

Investigation recordings

Site Temperature									
	Cold				Neutral				Hot
Atmosphere									
	Oppressive				Neutral				Light
Site observation									
Sensory Notes									

Equipment Used

Equipment	Readings

Investigation Date _____   Time _____

Address _____

Haunt Information

What happens?
Date of first experience
Description of events

Suspected entity information

Possible Names	Dates alive
Where entity lived	Entity's motives/wants
Story	

Investigation recordings

Site Temperature	Cold — Neutral — Hot
Atmosphere	Oppressive — Neutral — Light
Site observation	
Sensory Notes	

Equipment Used

Equipment	Readings

Investigation Date _____   Time _____

Address _____

Haunt Information

What happens?
Date of first experience
Description of events

Suspected entity information

Possible Names	Dates alive
Where entity lived	Entity's motives/wants
Story	

Investigation recordings

Site Temperature	Cold — Neutral — Hot	
Atmosphere	Oppressive — Neutral — Light	
Site observation		
Sensory Notes		

Equipment Used

Equipment	Readings

Investigation Date _____   Time _____

Address _____

Haunt Information

What happens?
Date of first experience
Description of events

Suspected entity information

Possible Names	Dates alive
Where entity lived	Entity's motives/wants
Story	

Investigation recordings

Site Temperature	Cold	Neutral	Hot
Atmosphere	Oppressive	Neutral	Light
Site observation			
Sensory Notes			

Equipment Used

Equipment	Readings

Investigation Date _____   Time _____

Address _____

Haunt Information

What happens?
Date of first experience
Description of events

Suspected entity information

Possible Names	Dates alive
Where entity lived	Entity's motives/wants
Story	

Investigation recordings

Site Temperature										
	Cold				Neutral					Hot
Atmosphere										
	Oppressive				Neutral					Light
Site observation										
Sensory Notes										

Equipment Used

Equipment	Readings

Investigation Date _____   Time _____

Address _____

Haunt Information

What happens?
Date of first experience
Description of events

Suspected entity information

Possible Names	Dates alive
Where entity lived	Entity's motives/wants
Story	

Investigation recordings

Site Temperature										
	Cold				Neutral					Hot
Atmosphere										
	Oppressive				Neutral					Light
Site observation										
Sensory Notes										

Equipment Used

Equipment	Readings

Investigation Date _____   Time _____

Address _____

Haunt Information

What happens?
Date of first experience
Description of events

Suspected entity information

Possible Names	Dates alive
Where entity lived	Entity's motives/wants
Story	

Investigation recordings

Site Temperature	Cold — Neutral — Hot
Atmosphere	Oppressive — Neutral — Light
Site observation	
Sensory Notes	

Equipment Used

Equipment	Readings

Investigation Date _____   Time _____

Address _____

Haunt Information

What happens?
Date of first experience
Description of events

Suspected entity information

Possible Names	Dates alive
Where entity lived	Entity's motives/wants
Story	

Investigation recordings

Site Temperature									
	Cold				Neutral				Hot
Atmosphere									
	Oppressive				Neutral				Light
Site observation									
Sensory Notes									

Equipment Used

Equipment	Readings

Investigation Date _____   Time _____

Address _____

Haunt Information

What happens?
Date of first experience
Description of events

Suspected entity information

Possible Names	Dates alive
Where entity lived	Entity's motives/wants
Story	

Investigation recordings

Site Temperature	Cold — Neutral — Hot
Atmosphere	Oppressive — Neutral — Light
Site observation	
Sensory Notes	

Equipment Used

Equipment	Readings

Investigation Date _____ Time _____

Address _____

Haunt Information

What happens?
Date of first experience
Description of events

Suspected entity information

Possible Names	Dates alive
Where entity lived	Entity's motives/wants
Story	

Investigation recordings

Site Temperature										
	Cold				Neutral					Hot
Atmosphere										
	Oppressive				Neutral					Light
Site observation										
Sensory Notes										

Equipment Used

Equipment	Readings

Investigation Date _____   Time _____

Address _____

Haunt Information

What happens?
Date of first experience
Description of events

Suspected entity information

Possible Names	Dates alive
Where entity lived	Entity's motives/wants
Story	

Investigation recordings

Site Temperature										
	Cold				Neutral					Hot
Atmosphere										
	Oppressive				Neutral					Light

Site observation

Sensory Notes

Equipment Used

Equipment	Readings

Investigation Date _____   Time _____

Address _____

Haunt Information

What happens?
Date of first experience
Description of events

Suspected entity information

Possible Names	Dates alive
Where entity lived	Entity's motives/wants
Story	

Investigation recordings

Site Temperature	Cold — Neutral — Hot
Atmosphere	Oppressive — Neutral — Light
Site observation	
Sensory Notes	

Equipment Used

Equipment	Readings

Investigation Date _____   Time _____

Address _____

Haunt Information

What happens?
Date of first experience
Description of events

Suspected entity information

Possible Names	Dates alive
Where entity lived	Entity's motives/wants
Story	

Investigation recordings

Site Temperature	Cold — Neutral — Hot
Atmosphere	Oppressive — Neutral — Light
Site observation	
Sensory Notes	

Equipment Used

Equipment	Readings

Investigation Date _____   Time _____

Address _____

Haunt Information

What happens?
Date of first experience
Description of events

Suspected entity information

Possible Names	Dates alive
Where entity lived	Entity's motives/wants
Story	

Investigation recordings

Site Temperature									
	Cold				Neutral				Hot
Atmosphere									
	Oppressive				Neutral				Light
Site observation									
Sensory Notes									

Equipment Used

Equipment	Readings

Investigation Date _____   Time _____

Address _____

Haunt Information

What happens?
Date of first experience
Description of events

Suspected entity information

Possible Names	Dates alive
Where entity lived	Entity's motives/wants
Story	

Investigation recordings

Site Temperature	Cold — Neutral — Hot
Atmosphere	Oppressive — Neutral — Light
Site observation	
Sensory Notes	

Equipment Used

Equipment	Readings

Investigation Date _____   Time _____

Address _____

Haunt Information

What happens?
Date of first experience
Description of events

Suspected entity information

Possible Names	Dates alive
Where entity lived	Entity's motives/wants
Story	

Investigation recordings

Site Temperature		
	Cold — Neutral — Hot	
Atmosphere		
	Oppressive — Neutral — Light	
Site observation		
Sensory Notes		

Equipment Used

Equipment	Readings

Investigation Date _____   Time _____

Address _____

Haunt Information

What happens?
Date of first experience
Description of events

Suspected entity information

Possible Names	Dates alive
Where entity lived	Entity's motives/wants
Story	

Investigation recordings

Site Temperature	Cold — Neutral — Hot
Atmosphere	Oppressive — Neutral — Light
Site observation	
Sensory Notes	

Equipment Used

Equipment	Readings

Investigation Date _____ Time _____

Address _____

Haunt Information

What happens?
Date of first experience
Description of events

Suspected entity information

Possible Names	Dates alive
Where entity lived	Entity's motives/wants
Story	

Investigation recordings

Site Temperature									
	Cold				Neutral				Hot
Atmosphere									
	Oppressive				Neutral				Light
Site observation									
Sensory Notes									

Equipment Used

Equipment	Readings

Investigation Date _____   Time _____

Address _____

Haunt Information

What happens?
Date of first experience
Description of events

Suspected entity information

Possible Names	Dates alive
Where entity lived	Entity's motives/wants
Story	

Investigation recordings

Site Temperature	Cold — Neutral — Hot
Atmosphere	Oppressive — Neutral — Light
Site observation	
Sensory Notes	

Equipment Used

Equipment	Readings

Investigation Date _____ Time _____

Address _____

Haunt Information

What happens?
Date of first experience
Description of events

Suspected entity information

Possible Names	Dates alive
Where entity lived	Entity's motives/wants
Story	

Investigation recordings

Site Temperature									
	Cold				Neutral				Hot
Atmosphere									
	Oppressive				Neutral				Light
Site observation									
Sensory Notes									

Equipment Used

Equipment	Readings

Investigation Date _____   Time _____

Address _____

Haunt Information

What happens?
Date of first experience
Description of events

Suspected entity information

Possible Names	Dates alive
Where entity lived	Entity's motives/wants
Story	

Investigation recordings

Site Temperature									
	Cold				Neutral				Hot

Atmosphere									
	Oppressive				Neutral				Light

Site observation

Sensory Notes

Equipment Used

Equipment	Readings

Investigation Date _____   Time _____

Address _____

Haunt Information

What happens?
Date of first experience
Description of events

Suspected entity information

Possible Names	Dates alive
Where entity lived	Entity's motives/wants
Story	

Investigation recordings

Site Temperature		
	Cold Neutral Hot	
Atmosphere		
	Oppressive Neutral Light	
Site observation		
Sensory Notes		

Equipment Used

Equipment	Readings

Investigation Date _____   Time _____

Address _____

Haunt Information

What happens?
Date of first experience
Description of events

Suspected entity information

Possible Names	Dates alive
Where entity lived	Entity's motives/wants
Story	

Investigation recordings

Site Temperature	Cold — Neutral — Hot	
Atmosphere	Oppressive — Neutral — Light	
Site observation		
Sensory Notes		

Equipment Used

Equipment	Readings

Investigation Date _____   Time _____

Address _____

Haunt Information

What happens?
Date of first experience
Description of events

Suspected entity information

Possible Names	Dates alive
Where entity lived	Entity's motives/wants
Story	

Investigation recordings

Site Temperature										
	Cold				Neutral					Hot
Atmosphere										
	Oppressive				Neutral					Light
Site observation										
Sensory Notes										

Equipment Used

Equipment	Readings

Investigation Date _____   Time _____

Address _____

Haunt Information

What happens?
Date of first experience
Description of events

Suspected entity information

Possible Names	Dates alive
Where entity lived	Entity's motives/wants
Story	

Investigation recordings

Site Temperature	Cold — Neutral — Hot
Atmosphere	Oppressive — Neutral — Light
Site observation	
Sensory Notes	

Equipment Used

Equipment	Readings

Investigation Date _____   Time _____

Address _____

Haunt Information

What happens?
Date of first experience
Description of events

Suspected entity information

Possible Names	Dates alive
Where entity lived	Entity's motives/wants
Story	

Investigation recordings

Site Temperature	Cold	Neutral	Hot
Atmosphere	Oppressive	Neutral	Light
Site observation			
Sensory Notes			

Equipment Used

Equipment	Readings

Investigation Date _____   Time _____

Address _____

Haunt Information

What happens?
Date of first experience
Description of events

Suspected entity information

Possible Names	Dates alive
Where entity lived	Entity's motives/wants
Story	

Investigation recordings

Site Temperature										
	Cold				Neutral					Hot
Atmosphere										
	Oppressive				Neutral					Light
Site observation										
Sensory Notes										

Equipment Used

Equipment	Readings

Investigation Date _____   Time _____

Address _____

Haunt Information

What happens?
Date of first experience
Description of events

Suspected entity information

Possible Names	Dates alive
Where entity lived	Entity's motives/wants
Story	

Investigation recordings

Site Temperature									
	Cold				Neutral				Hot
Atmosphere									
	Oppressive				Neutral				Light

Site observation

Sensory Notes

Equipment Used

Equipment	Readings

Investigation Date _____   Time _____

Address _____

Haunt Information

What happens?
Date of first experience
Description of events

Suspected entity information

Possible Names	Dates alive
Where entity lived	Entity's motives/wants
Story	

Investigation recordings

Site Temperature	Cold	Neutral	Hot
Atmosphere	Oppressive	Neutral	Light
Site observation			
Sensory Notes			

Equipment Used

Equipment	Readings

Investigation Date _____   Time _____

Address _____

Haunt Information

What happens?
Date of first experience
Description of events

Suspected entity information

Possible Names	Dates alive
Where entity lived	Entity's motives/wants
Story	

Investigation recordings

Site Temperature

Cold   Neutral   Hot

Atmosphere

Oppressive   Neutral   Light

Site observation

Sensory Notes

Equipment Used

Equipment	Readings

www.ingramcontent.com/pod-product-compliance
Lightning Source LLC
Chambersburg PA
CBHW071115030426
42336CB00013BA/2098